PENGUIN BOOKS

THE DIETER'S BIBLE

Muriel Kalish has been on and off countless diets for the
past twenty years. She lives in New York City.

THE
DIETER'S
BIBLE

365 WAYS
TO GET THEE
THROUGH
THE TOUGH
TIMES

MURIEL KALISH

PENGUIN BOOKS

PENGUIN BOOKS

Published by the Penguin Group

Penguin Books USA Inc., 375 Hudson Street,
New York, New York 10014, U.S.A.
Penguin Books Ltd, 27 Wrights Lane,
London W8 5TZ, England
Penguin Books Australia Ltd, Ringwood,
Victoria, Australia
Penguin Books Canada Ltd, 10 Alcorn Avenue,
Toronto, Ontario, Canada M4V 3B2
Penguin Books (N.Z.) Ltd, 182–190 Wairau Road,
Auckland 10, New Zealand

Penguin Books Ltd, Registered Offices:
Harmondsworth, Middlesex, England

First published in Penguin Books 1994

1 3 5 7 9 10 8 6 4 2

The product names used in this book that are known to be
trademarks appear in italics (e.g. *OREO*).

ISBN 0 14 01.7924 0

Printed in the United States of America
Set in Garamond
Design and illustration by Robert Clyde Anderson

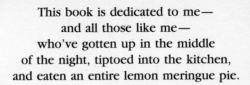

This book is dedicated to me—
and all those like me—
who've gotten up in the middle
of the night, tiptoed into the kitchen,
and eaten an entire lemon meringue pie.

INTRODUCTION

I began this book the night I crept out of bed, tiptoed into the kitchen, and—in total darkness—ate all the brownies my daughter and I had baked for her Christmas party at school. Depressed, disgusted, and more than a little queasy, I finally decided this sort of behavior was getting me nowhere. Yes, I was on a diet; yes, I wanted to lose weight—yet here I was at two in the morning eating every last crumb of my daughter's Christmas offering. Even going to my weight loss group wasn't helping. I'd come back from a meeting bursting with good intentions, but in a day or two everything I'd resolved went out of my head, while all sorts of fattening foods went into my mouth.

It dawned on me that what I really needed was a twenty-four-hour coach, a sort of buddy to keep me on track when the going got rough and that lemon meringue pie in the fridge was calling me by name. The next morning I taped two scraps of paper to my refrigerator. On one I'd written "Thou hast the courage to succeed" (I figured I'd pay more attention to it if it sounded like it came from a higher authority). The other said, "When thou canst not sleep, stay out of the kitchen!" As I was baking a make-up batch of brownies, I kept glancing up at my "commandments." They were wonderful reminders of what I was trying to accomplish. From that point on, I started writing down little "commandments" for myself, which I'd keep in my handbag, or stick on the bathroom mirror or in my desk at work. They really helped to keep me focused. To my great delight, they also became an instant hit with my friends and family—everyone wanted copies. And so it was at their urging that I put together this *Dieter's Bible*.

Let me say there's no special way to use this book—you can read through it or browse in it at will. But I hope you'll use it as you would a friend—someone who's there when you need that helping hand.

THE
DIETER'S
BIBLE

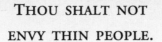

THOU SHALT NOT
ENVY THIN PEOPLE.

THOU SHALT RECOGNIZE
THAT COOKIES, CAKE, ICE CREAM,
AND CANDY ARE NOT
THE FOUR MAJOR FOOD GROUPS.

THOU SHALT NOT
EAT STANDING UP.

THOU SHALT HAVE
CONFIDENCE IN THYSELF.

THOU SHALT NOT
LIE ABOUT WHAT HAPPENED
TO THE DOUGHNUTS.

THOU SHALT START NOW.

THOU SHALT NOT
ADD UP HOW MANY DIETS
YOU HAVE BEEN ON
IN THE PAST.

THOU SHALT NOT
ENTER A SUPERMARKET
ON AN EMPTY STOMACH.

THOU SHALT REMEMBER
THAT FOOD EATEN
IN THE DARK COUNTS.

THOU SHALT HONOR
THY FATHER AND THY MOTHER
BY NOT EATING OFF THEIR PLATES.

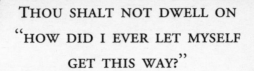

THOU SHALT NOT DWELL ON
"HOW DID I EVER LET MYSELF
GET THIS WAY?"

THOU SHALT FEEL GOOD
ABOUT YOURSELF EVERY TIME
YOU DON'T FINISH WHAT'S LEFT
IN THE BOTTOM OF THE POT.

THOU SHALT REALIZE IT'S POSSIBLE
TO HAVE COFFEE *WITHOUT* CAKE.

THOU SHALT LET YOUR BRAIN
BE AWARE OF WHAT
YOUR HANDS AND MOUTH ARE UP TO.

THOU SHALT CONTROL YOURSELF
—EVEN WHEN SOMEONE ELSE
IS PAYING FOR DINNER.

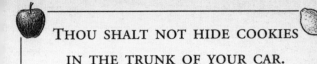

THOU SHALT NOT HIDE COOKIES
IN THE TRUNK OF YOUR CAR.

OR IN YOUR GLOVE
COMPARTMENT EITHER.

THOU HAST TRIUMPHED,
EVEN IF YOU HAVE ONLY:
1. SCRAPED THE WHIPPED CREAM
OFF THE BROWNIE.
2. LEFT SOME OF THE BROWNIE OVER.
3. NOT LICKED THE DISH.

THOU SHALT DRESS WELL,
NO MATTER WHAT YOUR WEIGHT.

THOU SHALT SAY TO YOURSELF
SIX TIMES A DAY:
"I DESERVE TO BE THINNER."

THOU SHALT NOT
EAT LEFTOVER LASAGNA
AT FOUR IN THE MORNING
BECAUSE YOU CAN'T SLEEP.

THOU SHALT BE ABLE
TO SIT THROUGH A MOVIE WITHOUT
GOING BACK FOR MORE POPCORN.

WHERE IS IT WRITTEN
THAT YOU MUST EAT
EVERYTHING ON YOUR PLATE?

OR FINISH EVERYTHING
IN THE PACKAGE?

THOU SHALT NOT COVET
OTHER PEOPLE'S FRENCH FRIES.

IF YOU HAVE TO LIE DOWN
AFTER YOU HAVE EATEN,
THOU HAST OVERDONE IT.

THOU SHALT LOOK FORWARD
TO NEVER AGAIN HAVING TO
RUMMAGE THROUGH THE CLOSET,
HOPING SOMETHING WILL FIT.

THOU SHALT LOVE THYSELF.

THOU SHALT NOT
PUSH THE SCALE ALL OVER
THE BATHROOM FLOOR,
TRYING TO GET A LOWER READING.

THOU SHALT LEARN
THE MAGIC WORDS—"I'M FULL."

THOU SHALT NOT TRY
TO TAKE IT ALL OFF AT ONCE—
ROME WASN'T BUILT IN A DAY,
AND NEITHER WERE YOUR HIPS.

IF YOU DO STRAY,
THOU SHALT NOT
BEAT UP ON YOURSELF.

THOU SHALT STOP USING FOOD
TO CALM YOUR FRAZZLED NERVES.

THOU SHALT NOT BLAME
BEN & JERRY'S FOR COMING OUT
WITH NEW FLAVORS.

THOU SHALT NOT EAT
REALLY FAST, AND THEN PICK
FOOD OFF YOUR HUSBAND'S PLATE.

THOU SHALT TALK BACK
"YOU KNOW THAT APPLE STRUDEL
TO YOURSELF:
YOU'VE BEEN THINKING ABOUT
ALL MORNING? *FORGET IT!*"

THOU SHALT AVOID
LICKING FOOD OFF YOUR FINGERS
(THAT GOES FOR
KNIVES AND BOWLS, TOO).

UNLESS YOU ARE DOING
SOMETHING NECESSARY, THOU SHALT
STAY OUT OF THE KITCHEN.

THOU SHALT KNOW THAT FOR YOU,
ONE NACHO IS TOO MANY—
A HUNDRED IS NOT ENOUGH.

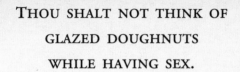

THOU SHALT NOT THINK OF
GLAZED DOUGHNUTS
WHILE HAVING SEX.

THOU SHALT EAT WITH DIGNITY:
AT THE TABLE, WITH A PLACEMAT
AND SILVERWARE—NOT AT THE SINK
WITH YOUR FINGERS.

THOU SHALT NOT
BE FRIENDS WITH ANYONE
WHO ONLY HAS PIZZA FOR LUNCH.

THOU SHALT BEWARE
OF FREE SAMPLES.

IF THOU SHOULDN'T EAT IT,
YOU SHOULDN'T HAVE IT
IN YOUR HANDBAG.

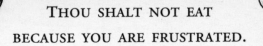

THOU SHALT NOT EAT
BECAUSE YOU ARE FRUSTRATED.

OR UNHAPPY.

OR HAPPY.

OR YOU HAVE GOTTEN A RAISE.

OR YOU HAVEN'T GOTTEN A RAISE.

OR YOUR BOYFRIEND DIDN'T CALL.

OR YOUR BOYFRIEND DID CALL.

OR YOU ARE VERY BUSY.

OR YOU HAVE NOTHING TO DO.

THOU SHALT ONLY EAT
BECAUSE THOU ART HUNGRY.

THOU SHALT NOT LET YOUR
MOTHER LOAD YOU UP WITH
GOODIES TO TAKE HOME.

IN A RESTAURANT,
THOU SHALT
NEVER UTTER THE WORDS,
"MORE BREAD, PLEASE."

FOOD SHALL BE
YOUR FRIEND—NOT YOUR ENEMY.

THOU SHALT NOT USE YOUR MOUTH
TO CLEAN UP AFTER DINNER.

THOU SHALT DO UNTO OTHERS
AS YOU WOULD HAVE THEM
DO UNTO YOU—SO DON'T
SERVE THEM PECAN PIE.

THOU SHALT NOT COMPARE
YOURSELF TO MADONNA OR CHER
(OR ANYONE ELSE
WITH A PERSONAL TRAINER).

THOU SHALT NOT HIDE CANDY BARS
UNDER YOUR SIDE OF THE MATTRESS.

THOU SHALT TAKE IT
ONE MEAL AT A TIME.

THOU SHALT NOT PATRONIZE
RESTAURANTS THAT SAY
"ALL YOU CAN EAT."

THOU SHALT REALIZE THAT
EATING CRUMBS (AND FROSTING
LEFT ON BOX COVERS) COUNTS.

THOU SHALT IGNORE PEOPLE
WHO SAY, "OH, YOU—YOU'RE
ALWAYS ON A DIET,"
OR "WHAT IS IT THIS TIME—
A GRAPEFRUIT A WEEK?"

THOU SHALT LEARN TO THROW AWAY
THE PACKAGE—EVEN IF
THERE ARE FOUR *FRITOS* LEFT.

THOU SHALT LOVE YOUR THIGHS.

THOU SHALT BE ABLE TO START
A DIET ANY DAY OF THE WEEK
—NOT JUST MONDAY.

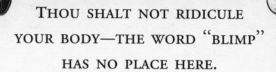

THOU SHALT NOT RIDICULE
YOUR BODY—THE WORD "BLIMP"
HAS NO PLACE HERE.

THOU SHALT BEWARE
OF PEOPLE SAYING,
"BUT I MADE IT JUST FOR *YOU!*"

THOU SHALT NOT
EAT YOUR KID'S LEFTOVERS.

IF IT'S TEMPTING,
THOU SHALT GET RID OF IT—
OUT OF SIGHT, OUT OF MOUTH.

THOU SHALT NOT
HIDE FOOD IN THE BOOKCASE.

THOU SHALT LET
YOUR CONSCIENCE BE YOUR GUIDE—
ESPECIALLY WHEN IT
COMES TO *OREOS*.

THOU SHALT NOT STARVE YOURSELF
BEFORE SHOPPING FOR A DRESS
AND STUFF YOURSELF
AFTER BUYING IT.

WHEN YOUR LITTLE
BLACK PARTY DRESS
WON'T FIT, THOU SHALT NOT
BLAME THE DRY CLEANER.

WHERE IS IT WRITTEN THAT BECAUSE
YOU GAVE UP SMOKING,
YOU MUST GAIN WEIGHT?

THOU SHALT KNOW THAT IN ALL
PROBABILITY THERE WILL *NOT* BE
A WORLDWIDE SHORTAGE OF COOKIES.

WHEN DRIVING, THOU SHALT NOT
EAT ANYTHING WHILE WAITING
FOR THE LIGHT TO CHANGE.

THOU SHALT REALIZE THAT
SUCCESS IS SAYING,
"I'LL KEEP TRYING."

FAILURE IS SAYING, "I GIVE UP."

DURING BUSINESS MEETINGS,
THOU SHALT TRY NOT TO THINK
ABOUT WHETHER THE DELI MAN
WILL REMEMBER TO PUT THE
COLESLAW ON THE SIDE.

THOU SHALT NOT BRING DIET
FOOD TO POTLUCK DINNERS—
AND THEN EAT EVERYTHING ELSE.

THOU SHALT REMEMBER:
PEACE OF MIND IS BETTER
THAN A PIECE OF CAKE.

THOU SHALT BEWARE
OF COCKTAIL PARTIES.

THOU SHALT NOT LET
ALL THOSE SKINNY YOUNG BODIES
AT THE HEALTH CLUB
GET YOU DOWN.

THOU ART EATING TOO FAST IF:
YOU ARE THE FIRST ONE DONE
AT ANY MEAL.

YOUR FORK ACTION IS A BLUR.

CHEWING IS SOMETHING
YOU HAVEN'T DONE MUCH OF
IN YEARS.

YOU ARE HELPING
OTHER PEOPLE FINISH THEIR FOOD.

YOU ARE ORDERING DESSERT
WHILE EVERYONE ELSE IS
STILL ON APPETIZERS.

THOU SHALT NOT REMINISCE
ABOUT WHAT YOU COULD EAT
IN THE GOOD OLD DAYS.

THOU SHALT LOOK FORWARD
TO SLEEVELESS DRESSES.

THOU SHALT NOT POLISH OFF
THE MEATLOAF, THE POTATOES,
AND THE TUNA FISH JUST SO
THEY WON'T SPOIL.

THOU SHALT IGNORE THE WORDS
"HOMEMADE ICE CREAM."

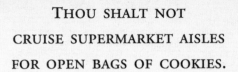

THOU SHALT NOT
CRUISE SUPERMARKET AISLES
FOR OPEN BAGS OF COOKIES.

THOU SHALT NOT
CRUISE SUPERMARKET AISLES
OPENING BAGS OF COOKIES.

THOU SHALT NOT
GET UPSET WHEN YOUR
HUSBAND DOESN'T NOTICE
YOU'VE LOST WEIGHT.

IF THOU ART BORED,
LIFE ISN'T MORE EXCITING
WHEN YOU'RE CHEWING *CHEETOS*.

THOU SHALT NOT
HAVE TOO MUCH OF ANYTHING
BECAUSE IT SMELLS SO GOOD.

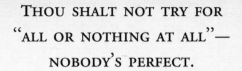

THOU SHALT NOT TRY FOR
"ALL OR NOTHING AT ALL"—
NOBODY'S PERFECT.

THOU SHALT NOT
"TEST YOUR WILLPOWER"
BY HAVING A LEMON MERINGUE PIE
IN THE REFRIGERATOR OVERNIGHT.

THOU SHALT NOT THINK
OF YOUR NEXT MEAL
THE MINUTE YOU'VE
FINISHED THE LAST ONE.

THOU SHALT HAVE
A POSITIVE ATTITUDE.

AT WORK, THOU SHALT NOT
HIDE CHOCOLATE IN YOUR DESK.

AND THOU SHALT NOT
DESTROY CANDY WRAPPER EVIDENCE
IN THE SHREDDER.

THOU SHALT REMEMBER THE
WORLD ISN'T ENDING TOMORROW,
SO YOU NEEDN'T EAT
ABSOLUTELY EVERYTHING *NOW*.

IT'S NOT FATE THAT DETERMINES
HOW MUCH GARLIC BREAD YOU EAT.

THOU SHALT NOT MAKE
UNREALISTIC PROMISES TO YOURSELF:
"I WILL NEVER EVEN *LOOK*
AT ANOTHER *ALMOND JOY*."

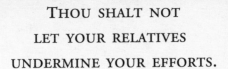

THOU SHALT NOT
LET YOUR RELATIVES
UNDERMINE YOUR EFFORTS.

THAT GOES FOR
YOUR CO-WORKERS TOO.

THOU SHALT WEAR SPANDEX
IF YOU REALLY WANT TO.

THOU SHALT NOT
BLAME THE HOLIDAYS.

THOU SHALT KNOW
THERE IS SUCH A THING
AS POPCORN *WITHOUT* BUTTER.

THOU SHALT NOT
ENGAGE IN OFFICE RIVALRIES
AS TO WHO LOSES WEIGHT FIRST.

OR WHO LOSES THE MOST.

THOU SHALT CONTROL YOUR FOOD
—NOT THE OTHER WAY AROUND.

BECAUSE THY LOVED ONES FORGOT
YOUR ANNIVERSARY IS NO REASON
TO GO THROUGH ALL THOSE
PISTACHIO NUTS.

THE WORD "SECONDS"
SHALL NOT BE IN THY VOCABULARY.

Thou shalt
make thy needs known to:
Your husband (or boyfriend).

Your mother.

Your mother-in-law.

Your friends.

Your children.

The waiter.

ON A DATE, THOU SHALT NOT
EAT PRACTICALLY NOTHING,
AND THEN GO HOME AND PIG OUT.

THOU SHALT LOVE YOUR BEHIND.

THOU SHALT NOT REWARD YOURSELF
WITH TORTILLA CHIPS
FOR CLEANING OUT THE DRAWERS.

THOU SHALT
LEARN TO TRUST YOURSELF.

IF YOUR ROOMMATE IS
A GOURMET COOK,
THOU SHALT CHANGE ROOMMATES.

THOU SHALT NOT MUNCH
PEANUT CHEWS JUST BECAUSE
THERE'S NOTHING GOOD ON TV.

THOU SHALT RECOGNIZE
THAT YOUR REFRIGERATOR IS NOT
THE CENTER OF THE UNIVERSE.

THOU SHALT THINK TWICE
ABOUT ANYTHING COVERED
WITH CHOCOLATE SPRINKLES

THOU SHALT SHOW
YOUR TASTE BUDS WHO'S BOSS.

THOU SHALT NOT KID YOURSELF
INTO BUYING *M & M'S* FOR THE KIDS
AND THEN EATING THEM YOURSELF.

THOU SHALT CHOOSE
BETWEEN COCONUT CREAM PIE
AND LOOKING GOOD IN SHORTS.

THOU SHALT NOT
EAT ANYTHING JUST BECAUSE
SOMEONE ELSE IS EATING IT.

THOU SHALT NOT THINK LESS
OF YOURSELF IF YOU CAN'T
HAVE PEANUT BUTTER IN THE HOUSE.

COOKBOOKS SHALL NOT BE
THY BEDTIME READING.

THOU SHALT NOT
EAT WITH ANYONE WHO CONSIDERS
FRIES AND A *COKE* A BALANCED MEAL.

THOU SHALT BELIEVE IN YOURSELF.

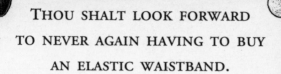

THOU SHALT LOOK FORWARD
TO NEVER AGAIN HAVING TO BUY
AN ELASTIC WAISTBAND.

OR AN OVERBLOUSE.

TO EAT CHOCOLATE
PUDDING IS HUMAN,
TO FORGIVE THYSELF DIVINE.

THOU SHALT ALWAYS ASK FOR
"THE DRESSING ON THE SIDE."

THOU SHALT NOT
LET AN EXPENSE ACCOUNT TURN
YOU INTO AN EATING MACHINE.

THOU SHALT NOT
HAVE BREAKFAST AT
TWO O'CLOCK IN THE MORNING
JUST BECAUSE YOU HAPPEN TO BE UP.

THOU SHALT NOT JUMP ON THE
SCALE EVERY FORTY-FIVE MINUTES.

THOU SHALT STOP SAYING "WHY ME?"

IF IT'S BEEN A BAD DAY,
THOU SHALT NOT UNWIND
WITH A JAR OF *CHEEZ WHIZ*.

WHEN THE CART COMES,
THOU SHALT NOT ENVY CO-WORKERS
WHO CAN HAVE COFFEE *AND* DANISH.

AT THE CHRISTMAS PARTY,
THOU ART NOT OBLIGED
TO *EAT*, DRINK, AND BE MERRY.

THE WORDS
"I DON'T CARE—I WANT IT!"
SHALL NEVER CROSS THY LIPS.

THOU SHALT NOT GET DISCOURAGED
BECAUSE YOUR JEANS
FROM TEN YEARS AGO WON'T FIT.

THOU SHALT DRIVE RIGHT PAST
ANY PLACE THAT ADVERTISES
"FRESHLY BAKED DOUGHNUTS."

THOU SHALT PRACTICE
MODERATION IN ALL THINGS,
ESPECIALLY COCKTAIL PEANUTS.

WHEN ENTERTAINING:
THOU SHALT NOT REGARD THIS
AS YOUR CHANCE TO GO BERSERK.

DO NOT PREPARE FORBIDDEN FOODS
FOR THY GUESTS,
JUST SO YOU CAN EAT
THE LEFTOVERS WHEN THEY LEAVE.

THOU SHALT MAKE FOOD
THAT'S GOOD FOR *YOU* TO EAT.

AND THOU SHALT NOT
GO OVERBOARD ON DESSERTS.
THOU SHALT SERVE FRUIT
OR FROZEN YOGURT (OR ANYTHING
ELSE THAT'S LIGHT AND HEALTHY).

AS FOR CLEARING THE TABLE,
DO *NOT* DO THIS BY YOURSELF—
ASK FOR HELP. OR
(IF YOU ARE NOT TOO
ELEGANT FOR THIS)
HAVE EVERYONE THROW OUT THEIR
OWN GARBAGE.

AND WHEN THEY'RE LEAVING,
MAKE SURE YOUR
GUESTS TAKE HOME WHATEVER
TEMPTING THINGS ARE LEFT.

THOU HAST EATEN TOO MUCH
IF AFTER A MEAL
YOU NEVER WANT TO EAT AGAIN.

THOU SHALT BREAK NEW GROUND:
A WAFFLE *WITHOUT* SYRUP.

THOU SHALT AVOID PESSIMISTIC
GRUMPS WHO FEEL THEY
CAN'T DIET AND NEITHER CAN YOU.

THOU NEEDN'T BE OVERWEIGHT
—IT'S NOT WRITTEN IN THE STARS,
ONLY ON YOUR SHOPPING LIST.

WHEN YOU FEEL
A BINGE COMING ON, THOU SHALT
GET OUT OF THE KITCHEN.

THOU SHALT NOT
USE GETTING MARRIED AS
AN EXCUSE FOR GAINING WEIGHT.

THOU SHALT NOT
USE GETTING DIVORCED AS
AN EXCUSE FOR GAINING WEIGHT.

THOU SHALT THINK TWICE
ABOUT ANY FRIEND WHO INVITES
YOU TO A LOW CALORIE DINNER—
AND THEN SERVES LASAGNA,
FRENCH BREAD, AND BROWNIES.

THOU SHALT BE
YOUR OWN CHEERLEADER.

IN SUPERMARKETS,
THOU SHALT AVOID ANY AISLE
THAT MAKES YOU SALIVATE.

THOU SHALT REALIZE THAT
BY THE TIME A CROISSANT IS IN
YOUR HAND, IT'S USUALLY TOO LATE.

THOU SHALT PUT REMINDERS
TO YOURSELF ON YOUR
REFRIGERATOR DOOR.

AND YOUR KITCHEN CABINETS.

AND ANYWHERE ELSE
YOU CAN THINK OF.

IF THY HUSBAND INSISTS
ON KEEPING FUDGE IN THE HOUSE,
THOU SHALT ASSERT YOURSELF.

THOU SHALT NOT GO OUT
AT THREE IN THE MORNING LOOKING
FOR A PIZZA PARLOR THAT'S OPEN.

THOU SHALT COOK
NORMAL PORTIONS.

THOU SHALT NOT HIDE FOOD
IN THE WASHING MACHINE.

THOU SHALT REMEMBER
YOU HAVE THE POWER
TO MAKE CHOICES.

THOU SHALT NEVER SAY,
"HOW COULD I HAVE EATEN *THAT*?"
(WE'VE ALL EATEN
FROZEN *SARA LEE* POUND CAKE).

THOU SHALT NOT CONTINUE
SEEING ANYONE WHO ENCOURAGES
YOU TO EAT AND THEN
COMPLAINS ABOUT YOUR HIPS.

THOU SHALT EXERCISE.

THOU SHALT NOT REWARD YOURSELF
WITH A HOT FUDGE SUNDAE
AFTER EXERCISING.

THOU SHALT TELL THAT LITTLE VOICE
IN YOUR HEAD THAT WHISPERS
"HOW ABOUT A *RING DING*?"
TO GET LOST.

THOU SHALT REMEMBER
THAT A LITTLE NIBBLE HERE AND
A LITTLE NIBBLE THERE DO ADD UP.

FOR HALLOWEEN TRICK-OR-TREATING,
THOU SHALT BUY ONLY
THE CANDY YOU HATE.

BETTER STILL,
THOU SHALT GIVE OUT NOISE-MAKERS,
BALLOONS, OR PENNIES INSTEAD.

AND ABOVE ALL,
THOU SHALT NOT EAT
THE STUFF YOUR KID BRINGS HOME.

On a date, if thou art thinking only of the peanut butter and marshmallow sandwich you'll whip up at home, this is not the mate for you.

Thou shalt not put off swimming or skiing or dancing (or sex, for that matter) until you are thinner.

Thou shalt not blame your glands.

If you shouldn't be eating it, thou shalt not bring it into the house.

THOU SHALT REWARD THYSELF
FOR EATING RIGHT.
SO GET YOURSELF A MANICURE.

OR BUY SOME EARRINGS.

OR READ SOMETHING WONDERFUL.

OR CALL AN OLD FRIEND
WHO LIVES FAR AWAY.

OR GIVE YOURSELF
A LONG-STEMMED ROSE.

THOU SHALT NOT GRAB
A HANDFUL OF FRIES OFF YOUR
BOYFRIEND'S PLATE AND
THINK IT DOESN'T COUNT.

THOU SHALT LOVE YOUR UPPER ARMS.

THOU SHALT LOOK FORWARD
TO NOT AVOIDING PEOPLE
WHO KNEW YOU IN HIGH SCHOOL
WHEN YOU WERE A LOT THINNER.

WHEN GIVEN A MENU,
THOU SHALT NOT TURN TO
THE DESSERTS FIRST.

THOU SHALT FEEL GOOD
ABOUT YOURSELF EVERY TIME
YOU HAVE A CARROT
INSTEAD OF A COOKIE.

THOU SHALT NOT HANDLE STRESS
WITH BANANA NUT CAKE.

THOU SHALT NOT USE
YOUR REFRIGERATOR FOR BROWSING.
TAKE WHAT YOU WANT—AND *LEAVE*.

"WHY NOT HAVE IT JUST THIS ONCE,"
SHALT GO IN ONE EAR
AND OUT THE OTHER.

THOU SHALT NOT
EAT TUNA FISH EVERY SINGLE DAY.

IN FACT, NO MATTER WHAT IT IS,
THOU SHALT NOT EAT IT
EVERY SINGLE DAY.

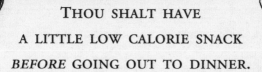

THOU SHALT HAVE
A LITTLE LOW CALORIE SNACK
BEFORE GOING OUT TO DINNER.

THOU SHALT THINK
OF YOUR DIET AS A CHALLENGE.

THOU SHALT NEVER PICK UP
A COOKBOOK WHEN YOU ARE HUNGRY.

IF THE BOX SAYS "SUPER RICH,"
THOU SHALT PUT IT BACK.

THOU SHALT GET RIGHT BACK ON
YOUR DIET—EVEN THOUGH YOU JUST
HAD LAST NIGHT'S COLD SPAGHETTI
AND A WHOLE JAR OF OLIVES.

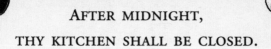

AFTER MIDNIGHT,
THY KITCHEN SHALL BE CLOSED.

THOU SHALT NOT KID THYSELF
INTO THINKING YOU CAN HAVE
JUST *ONE* PEANUT.

THOU SHALT REMEMBER:
DRINKS HAVE CALORIES.

THOU SHALT KNOW IT'S ACTUALLY
POSSIBLE TO GO THROUGH THE MALL
WITHOUT EATING ANYTHING.

THOU SHALT GET OUT OF
TROUBLESOME SITUATIONS
BEFORE IT'S TOO LATE.

THOU SHALT NOT LOSE WEIGHT
FOR OTHERS—THIS IS FOR YOU.

THOU SHALT NOT AVOID
FULL LENGTH MIRRORS.

THAT GOES FOR
THREE-WAY MIRRORS TOO.

THOU SHALT NOT EAT
AS IF THIS IS YOUR LAST MEAL.

IT'S A BAD SIGN IF
THEY KNOW YOU BY YOUR FIRST NAME
AT *DUNKIN' DONUTS*.

IF THY FRIENDSHIP
IS BASED ON EATING,
YOU WILL FIND A NEW FRIEND.

TIGHT JEANS ARE NATURE'S WAY
OF SAYING THOU OVERDID IT.

THOU SHALT THINK BEFORE YOU EAT
(ESPECIALLY AT BUFFETS).

THOU SHALT NOT SNEAK *SNICKERS*
INTO THE LADIES' ROOM.

THOU SHALT COMPLIMENT OTHERS
WHEN THEY LOSE WEIGHT.

THE FOLLOWING
SHALT NOT ENTER YOUR MIND:
"I'LL START TOMORROW."

"IT'S JUST NO USE."

"I'M TOO OLD TO DIET."

"I MAY AS WELL
FINISH UP THE REST."

"I'M SUCH A FAILURE."

"BOY, COULD I USE
A CHEESEBURGER."

THOU SHALT STOP
BLAMING YOUR MOTHER FOR NOT
TEACHING YOU TO EAT RIGHT.

IF YOU HAVE A FRIEND
WITH THE SAME PROBLEM,
THOU SHALT BE THERE FOR HER
(AND VICE VERSA).

THOU SHALT BEWARE LEST
"STRESSED OUT" LEAD TO "PIG OUT."

THOU SHALT KEEP
A SMALL-SIZE DRESS AROUND
AS A REMINDER OF YOUR GOAL.

WHEN FACE-TO-FACE
WITH PEANUT BRITTLE,
THOU SHALT BE STRONG.

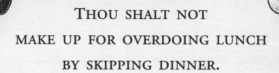

THOU SHALT NOT
MAKE UP FOR OVERDOING LUNCH
BY SKIPPING DINNER.

THOU SHALT GIVE YOURSELF
THE GIFT OF LOOKING BETTER.

THOU SHALT REST
WHEN YOU ARE TIRED,
NOT EAT "FOR ENERGY."

THOU SHALT NOT HIDE FOOD
IN THE BABY'S STROLLER.

THOU SHALT KEEP IN MIND
THAT EATING A BLUEBERRY PIE
WILL NOT MAKE YOU
ANY LESS ANGRY AT YOUR HUSBAND.

THOU SHALT TELL YOURSELF
HOW WONDERFUL YOU ARE
AT LEAST ONCE A DAY.

THOU SHALT NOT
EAT A LOT *NOW*, JUST IN CASE
YOU MIGHT GET HUNGRY *LATER*.

THOU SHALT KEEP A RECORD
OF WHAT YOU EAT—
IT REALLY DOES HELP.

THOU SHALT NOT SNATCH LUNCH
ON THE WAY TO
YOUR NEXT APPOINTMENT.

THOU SHALT HAVE GREAT SEX
—IT'LL TAKE YOUR MIND OFF FOOD.

THOU SHALT NOT FEEL DEPRIVED
WHEN YOU CAN'T HAVE
THE ENTIRE PINT
OF ROCKY ROAD ICE CREAM.

THOU SHALT REALIZE
THAT WHAT FOLLOWS A BINGE
IS NOT CONTENTMENT
BUT ANOTHER BINGE.

THOU SHALT NOT GET UPSET
WHEN YOUR MOTHER-IN-LAW SAYS,
"DIDN'T THEY HAVE THAT BLOUSE
IN YOUR SIZE?"

THOU SHALT NOT POLISH OFF
YOUR KID'S ANIMAL CRACKERS.

THOU SHALT AVOID
EATING WHILE STANDING IN FRONT
OF AN OPEN REFRIGERATOR.

THOU SHALT REMEMBER
IT'S *YOUR* MOUTH—NO ONE ELSE
CAN DECIDE WHAT GOES IN IT.

THOU SHALT NOT SEND OUT FOR
TWO PIZZAS AT A TIME JUST BECAUSE
IT'S CHEAPER THAT WAY.

THOU SHALT LOVE YOUR HIPS.

THOU SHALT NOT
PUT IN A NEW MOUTHFUL
UNTIL THE LAST ONE'S FINISHED.

THOU SHALT NOT
REWARD THYSELF WITH
TWO APPLE TURNOVERS
FOR CALLING YOUR MOTHER.

THOU SHALT BE OPTIMISTIC.

AFTER OVEREATING,
THOU SHALT NOT PUNISH YOURSELF
BY EATING EVEN MORE.

THOU SHALT SHUN
FOODS DESCRIBED AS "FUDGY."

WHEN IN CHINESE RESTAURANTS,
THOU SHALT GO EASY
ON THE CRISPY NOODLES.

THOU SHALT MAKE A LIST OF
ALTERNATIVES TO GOING ON A BINGE:
LIKE TAKING A WALK.

OR RENTING SOME GREAT VIDEOS.

OR BROWSING THROUGH
YOUR FAVORITE CLOTHING STORE.

OR STARTING A DIARY.

OR ANYTHING ELSE THAT GRABS YOU.

THOU SHALT NOT EAT IT
BECAUSE NOBODY ELSE WANTS IT.

THOU SHALT NOT BE
A MAYONNAISE ABUSER.

THOU SHALT TRY TO KEEP CALM
AT THE SIGHT OF A BAKERY.

OR THE SOUND
OF A CANDY WRAPPER BEING OPENED.

OR THE SMELL OF FRENCH FRIES.

THOU SHALT NOT
HAVE A LOVE-HATE RELATIONSHIP
WITH FOOD.

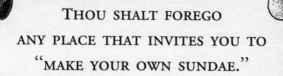

THOU SHALT FOREGO
ANY PLACE THAT INVITES YOU TO
"MAKE YOUR OWN SUNDAE."

IF THOU ABSOLUTELY MUST,
BETTER ONE VANILLA WAFER
THAN THE WHOLE PACKAGE.

AS FOR THE STRAWBERRY SHORTCAKE,
THOU SHALT NOT CLAIM
THE DOG ATE IT.

THOU SHALT REMIND YOURSELF
—WHEN YOU ARE COOKING,
TASTING COUNTS.

THOU SHALT FIND SOMETHING
TO READ BESIDES YOUR SCALE.

THOU SHALT NOT DEPEND
ON SOMEONE ELSE TO STOP YOU
BEFORE YOU TAKE ANOTHER BITE.

THOU SHALT HAVE A GREAT HAIRDO,
NO MATTER WHAT YOU WEIGH.

THOU SHALT NOT WASTE ENERGY
FEELING GUILTY (EVEN IF YOU
ATE UP LAST NIGHT'S RAVIOLI,
ALL THE BREAD IN THE HOUSE,
AND SOMETHING FROM THE BACK OF
THE REFRIGERATOR YOU COULDN'T
QUITE IDENTIFY).

THOU SHALT SKIP
ANY PART OF THE MALL
THAT SMELLS TOO GOOD.

THOU SHALT NOT FEEL SELFISH
FOR FOCUSING ON YOURSELF.

THOU SHALT TRY
WATCHING TV *WITHOUT* EATING.

THOU SHALT HAVE POWER
OVER YOUR KNIFE AND FORK.

THOU SHALT NO LONGER BE
AN EXTREMIST—IT DOESN'T HAVE TO
BE EITHER FOUR STRINGBEANS
OR AN ENTIRE BOSTON CREAM PIE.

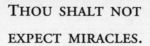

THOU SHALT NOT
EXPECT MIRACLES.

THOU SHALT KEEP
FRUIT AND VEGETABLES HANDY.

THOU SHALT NOT USE
SPECIAL OCCASIONS AS AN EXCUSE
TO PIG OUT.

THOU SHALT LOOK FORWARD
TO THE EXPRESSION
ON YOUR SISTER-IN-LAW'S FACE
WHEN SHE SEES YOU
LOOKING SO GREAT!

THOU SHALT NOT EAT
AS IF ON FAST FORWARD.

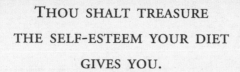

THOU SHALT TREASURE
THE SELF-ESTEEM YOUR DIET
GIVES YOU.

THOU SHALT NOT HIDE FOOD
IN THE FILING CABINET.

THOU SHALT LEARN TO SAY "NO"
(TO OTHERS AND TO *YOURSELF*).

IF YOUR HOBBY IS BAKING,
THOU SHALT GET ANOTHER HOBBY.

THOU SHALT EXPECT
THE BEST FROM YOURSELF.

"TO SEE IT IS TO EAT IT,"
SHALL NO LONGER BE THY CREED.

IF THOU ART
INVITED TO DINNER,
AND YOUR HOSTESS ISN'T HELPFUL,
THERE ARE ALTERNATIVES:
FOR INSTANCE,
BRING YOUR OWN FOOD
(THIS IS NOT AS TOUGH
AS IT SOUNDS).

YOU COULD BRING A FROZEN DINNER
AND PUT IT IN YOUR HOSTESS' OVEN
(OR MICROWAVE).

OR YOU COULD BRING SOME
COLD STUFF IN PLASTIC CONTAINERS.

OR IF ALL ELSE FAILS,
YOU COULD MAKE A DATE THAT
DOESN'T INVOLVE EATING.

WHEN YOU CAN'T SLEEP,
THOU SHALT NOT COUNT
PEANUT BUTTER CUPS.

THOU SHALT STOP WONDERING
HOW COME TEENAGERS CAN EAT
ALL THEY WANT AND
NOT GAIN A POUND.

THOU SHALT NOT FEEL
YOU MUST EAT *ALL* THE FOOD
YOU BROUGHT ON A PICNIC,
JUST SO YOU NEEDN'T TAKE IT HOME.

IF LUNCH AT WORK IS A PROBLEM,
THOU SHALT BROWN-BAG IT.

THOU SHALT LOVE YOUR TUMMY.

THOU SHALT AVOID
ANY RECIPE CALLING FOR
A PINT OF WHIPPING CREAM.

THOU SHALT SELECT A ROLE MODEL
—SOMEONE WHO'S LOST WEIGHT
AND KEPT IT OFF.

THY FANTASIES SHALL BE CONCERNED
WITH SEX, NOT *MALLOMARS*.

THOU SHALT REMEMBER:
HALF A DIET IS BETTER THAN NONE.

THOU SHALT MAKE FRIENDS
WITH BROCCOLI.

IF DINNER AT YOUR MOM'S
IS TOO MUCH OF A STRAIN,
THOU SHALT VISIT *AFTER* MEALS.

THOU SHALT ASK FOR HELP.

THOU SHALT AVOID CO-WORKERS
WHO KEEP OPEN COOKIE BOXES
ON THEIR DESKS.

THOU SHALT STOP
DOUBTING YOURSELF.

THOU SHALT NOT EAT ANYTHING
BECAUSE SOMEONE ELSE
WANTS YOU TO.

THOU SHALT REMEMBER
THAT *TOOTSIE ROLLS* HAVE
NO REAL POWER OVER YOU.

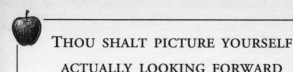

THOU SHALT PICTURE YOURSELF
ACTUALLY LOOKING FORWARD
TO GOING TO THE BEACH.

THOU SHALT NOT BLAME
YOUR LOVED ONES IF THEY CAN
EAT MORE THAN YOU DO
WITHOUT GAINING WEIGHT.

THOU SHALT RESPECT YOURSELF.

THOU SHALT NOT THINK
YOURSELF WEIRD IF YOU TAKE
AN APPLE EVERYWHERE YOU GO.

THOU SHALT NOT SEEK
EMPLOYMENT IN PIZZA PARLORS
AND DOUGHNUT SHOPS.

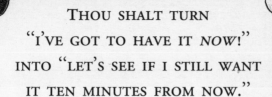

THOU SHALT TURN
"I'VE GOT TO HAVE IT *NOW!*"
INTO "LET'S SEE IF I STILL WANT
IT TEN MINUTES FROM NOW."

THOU ART NEITHER
GOOD NOR BAD BECAUSE
YOU HAD POTATOES AU GRATIN.

THOU SHALT NOT FIND
A WAY TO EAT WHILE EXERCISING.

IF YOU GET MAD
AT YOUR BOSS, THOU
SHALT NOT PUNISH HIM
BY HAVING *FIG NEWTONS.*

THOU SHALT NOT HAVE A DANISH
BEFORE AEROBICS AND THEN FEEL
YOU WORKED IT OFF.

THOU SHALT AVOID THE KITCHEN
WHEN YOU ARE ALL STRESSED OUT.

THOU SHALT NOT LET YOUR DIET
TURN YOU INTO A GROUCH.

THOU SHALT NOT COMPLAIN
TO EVERYONE YOU KNOW
ABOUT LOSING WEIGHT TOO SLOWLY.

THOU SHALT NOT
EAT MORE BETWEEN MEALS
THAN YOU EAT *AT* MEALS.

IF YOU ARE THINKING
OF MACARONI AND CHEESE
WHILE READING A THRILLER,
THOU SHALT CHANGE THRILLERS.

THOU SHALT TAKE
RESPONSIBILITY FOR YOURSELF.

THOU SHALT NOT FOCUS
ON ALL THE THINGS YOU CAN'T EAT
(THINK OF ALL THE THINGS
YOU *CAN* EAT).

THOU SHALT STOP
WONDERING WHY EVERYTHING
THAT TASTES GOOD IS BAD.

THOU SHALT BEWARE
OF *HORS D'OEUVRES*.

THOU SHALT NOT UPSET THYSELF
WITH THOUGHTS LIKE
"MY HUSBAND'S
LOOKING AT SKINNY WOMEN."

OR "I'LL BE THE FATTEST ONE
IN THAT WHOLE AEROBICS CLASS."

OR "I CAN'T GO TO THE REUNION
—NOBODY WILL RECOGNIZE ME."

OR "MY BOYFRIEND WON'T WANT
TO KEEP THE LIGHTS ON ANYMORE."

THOU SHALT THINK POSITIVE
THOUGHTS.

THOU SHALT NOT EAT
SOMETHING YOU SHOULDN'T
AND THEN HIDE THE WRAPPER
IN THE BOTTOM OF THE GARBAGE.

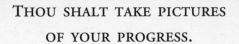

THOU SHALT TAKE PICTURES
OF YOUR PROGRESS.

THOU SHALT NEVER
EAT FROM A SAUCEPAN.

THOU SHALT ACCEPT
COMPLIMENTS GRACEFULLY.

THOU SHALT FORGET
WHAT YOUR MOTHER USED TO SAY
ABOUT WASTING FOOD
(YOU AREN'T HELPING CONDITIONS
IN INDIA BY EATING *OREOS*).

THOU HAST THE
COURAGE TO SUCCEED.

WHILE DINING WITH FRIENDS,
THOU SHALT THINK OF SOMETHING
BESIDES DESSERT.

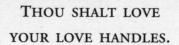

THOU SHALT LOVE
YOUR LOVE HANDLES.

THOU SHALT NOT HAVE
A FUDGE BROWNIE
IN THE AFTERNOON
AND THEN DECIDE,
"THAT WAS DINNER."

THOU SHALT ATTEMPT
THE UNKNOWN —
A MOVIE *WITHOUT* CANDY.

THOU SHALT NOT START EATING
FOODS YOU CAN'T *STOP* EATING.

THE PHRASE
"HAND-DIPPED CHOCOLATE"
SHALL HAVE NO PLACE
IN YOUR THOUGHTS.

THOU SHALT NOT SNEAK
INTO THE KITCHEN AT
THREE IN THE MORNING AND
EAT BY THE REFRIGERATOR LIGHT.

THOU SHALT NOTICE
HOW SLOWLY SOME PEOPLE EAT.

THOU SHALT REMEMBER
—NOBODY'S EVER DIED
FROM NOT HAVING
CHOCOLATE COVERED ALMONDS.

THOU SHALT BE AWARE
THAT IF YOU FAIL TO PREPARE,
YOU PREPARE TO FAIL.

IF YOU HAVE TO HIDE IT,
THOU SHALT NOT EAT IT.

UNLESS YOUR MOTHER'S BUILT
LIKE THE INCREDIBLE HULK,
THOU SHALT NOT BLAME
"BIG BONES" FOR YOUR PROBLEM.

THOU SHALT REMEMBER,
"TO THINE OWN SELF BE TRUE"
(EXCEPT WHEN YOU WANT A MALTED).

THOU SHALT HONOR THY BODY,
NO MATTER WHAT IT LOOKS LIKE
RIGHT NOW.

AND THOU SHALT FOCUS
ON WHAT IT *WILL* LOOK LIKE.

AND IF THOU HAST GONE OVERBOARD,
YOU SHALL FORGIVE YOURSELF,
AND START AGAIN.